I0702934

A COMPLETE GUIDE TO GUASHA SCRAPPING TECHNIQUE

The Complete Guide To Natural Way Of Prevention And Treatment Through Traditional Chinese Medicine Everything You Need To Know About Gua Sha

Faith Lynch

Table of Contents

INTRODUCTION TO GUASHA 2

A. Overview Of Guasha 2

Definition And Pronunciation 2

Brief History And Origins 2

B. Importance In Traditional Chinese Medicine (Tcm).............2

Role In Holistic Health Practices 2

Modern Relevance And Resurgence 2

A. Overview of Gua Sha 2

B. Importance in Traditional Chinese Medicine (TCM) 5

CHAPTER ONE 9

HISTORICAL CONTEXT 9

A. Origins And Evolution 9

Ancient China: Early Practices And Philosophies 9

Development Through Dynasties (Han, Tang, Ming, Qing)......9

B. Influences And Adaptations...9

Impact On Neighboring Cultures (Korea, Japan, Vietnam) 9

Integration Into Western Practices..9

1. Ancient China: Early Practices and Philosophies 9

2. Development Through Dynasties...11

B. Influences and Adaptations 14

2. Integration into Western Practices......................................17

THE THEORY BEHIND GUASHA..20

A. Traditional Chinese Medicine Principles............................20

Qi (Energy) And Blood Flow 20

Meridian Systems And Acupoints 20

B. Guasha Tools And Techniques 20

Materials Used (Jade, Horn, Plastic, Etc.) 20

Common Techniques And Their Purposes 20

A. Traditional Chinese Medicine Principles.........................20

B. Gua Sha Tools and Techniques 25

CHAPTER TWO 32

THE PRACTICE OF GUASHA 32

A. Preparing For Guasha 32

Setting Up The Environment...32

Choosing Appropriate Tools And Techniques.......................32

B. Step-By-Step Guide 32

Detailed Instructions For Self-Care 32

Professional Practice And What To Expect............................32

C. Common Areas Of Application 32

Neck And Shoulders...32

Back And Legs 32

Face And Scalp 32

A. Preparing for Gua Sha..32

B. Step-by-Step Guide 36

C. Common Areas of Application 41

BENEFITS AND EFFECTS 45

A. Physiological Benefits 45

Improved Circulation 45

Pain Relief And Muscle Relaxation 45

B. Psychological And Emotional Benefits............................45

Stress Reduction 45

Enhanced Overall Well-Being 45

C. Case Studies And Anecdotes......................................45

Personal Stories And Testimonials..................................45

Clinical Observations And Research Findings 45

A. Physiological Benefits 45

B. Psychological and Emotional Benefits 49

C. Case Studies and Anecdotes.......................................51

CHAPTER THREE 55

ADDRESSING MISCONCEPTIONS.....................................55

A. Myths Vs. Facts..55

Common Misconceptions Debunked................................55

Evidence-Based Clarifications 55

B. Potential Risks And Precautions 55

Safety Guidelines 55

Contraindications And When To Avoid............................55

A. Myths vs. Facts 55

B. Potential Risks and Precautions..................................61

INTEGRATION WITH MODERN PRACTICES 64

A. Guasha In Contemporary Wellness 64

Usage In Spas And Wellness Centers 64

Integration With Other Therapies (Acupuncture, Massage) .64

B. Guasha In Daily Life...64

Incorporating Into A Wellness Routine................................64

Adaptations For Different Lifestyles And Needs....................64

A. Gua Sha in Contemporary Wellness 64

B. Gua Sha in Daily Life 70

CHAPTER FOUR 75

CULTURAL AND PERSONAL REFLECTIONS................75

A. Guasha In Personal Journeys 75

Personal Reflections And Transformations.......................75

Stories From Practitioners And Patients 75

B. Cultural Significance 75

Symbolism And Cultural Narratives 75

Guasha's Role In Preserving Cultural Heritage 75

A. Gua Sha in Personal Journeys................................75

B. Cultural Significance 80

FUTURE DIRECTIONS...85

A. Evolving Practices And Research 85

Emerging Trends And Innovations.............................85

Ongoing Research And Studies 85

B. Expanding Awareness 85

Educational Initiatives And Workshops 85

Global Recognition And Acceptance...........................85

A. Evolving Practices and Research.............................85

B. Expanding Awareness 90

CONCLUSION 95

A. Summary Of Key Points 95

Recap Of Guasha's Significance And Benefits.......................95

B. Final Thoughts 95

Encouragement For Readers To Explore And Experience Guasha 95

A. Summary of Key Points..95

B. Final Thoughts 99

END 102

INTRODUCTION TO GUASHA

A. Overview Of Guasha

Definition And Pronunciation

Brief History And Origins

B. Importance In Traditional Chinese Medicine (Tcm)

Role In Holistic Health Practices

Modern Relevance And Resurgence

A. Overview of Gua Sha

1. Definition and Pronunciation

Definition: Gua Sha (pronounced "gwah-shah") is a traditional Chinese healing technique that involves scraping the skin with a smooth-edged tool to improve circulation, alleviate pain, and promote overall health. The term "Gua" means to scrape or rub, and "Sha" refers to the redness or minor bruising that appears on the skin after the treatment. The technique often uses tools made from materials like jade, quartz, or stainless steel.

Pronunciation: Gua Sha is pronounced as "gwah-shah," with "Gua" sounding like "gwa" and "Sha" sounding like "shah."

2. Brief History and Origins

Origins: Gua Sha has deep roots in Chinese history and is believed to date back thousands of years. Its origins can be traced to traditional Chinese practices where it was used for various health benefits, such as treating fevers and improving overall vitality.

Historical Use: Ancient Chinese texts and records suggest that Gua Sha was used by practitioners to address issues related to the body's qi (vital energy) and blood flow. Over time, it became an integral part of Traditional Chinese Medicine (TCM) due to its effectiveness in treating a range of ailments.

Evolution: Traditionally, Gua Sha was performed using everyday items such as spoons or coins, but as the practice evolved, specific tools were developed. Today, it is practiced both in traditional settings and modern health practices, with variations in techniques and tools.

B. Importance in Traditional Chinese Medicine (TCM)

1. Role in Holistic Health Practices

TCM Principles: In Traditional Chinese Medicine, Gua Sha is used based on the principle that health is maintained through balanced qi (energy flow) and blood circulation. By scraping the skin, Gua Sha aims to release stagnation, improve circulation, and promote healing.

Holistic Approach: TCM views health as a balance between various bodily systems and external factors. Gua Sha is used to address imbalances and support the body's natural healing processes. It is often employed alongside other TCM practices like acupuncture, herbal medicine, and cupping.

Therapeutic Uses: Practitioners use Gua Sha to treat a variety of conditions, including muscle pain, tension, respiratory issues, and digestive problems. The technique is believed to help with muscle relaxation, reduce inflammation, and enhance immune function.

2. Modern Relevance and Resurgence

Increased Popularity: In recent years, Gua Sha has seen a resurgence in popularity beyond traditional Chinese settings. It is increasingly recognized and utilized in Western wellness and holistic health practices.

Scientific Support: Modern research has started to validate some of the benefits of Gua Sha, such as its effects on pain relief and circulation. While more research is needed, preliminary studies suggest that Gua Sha may help reduce muscle soreness and improve circulation.

Adaptations: The practice has been adapted and integrated into modern health and beauty routines. For instance, Gua Sha tools are now commonly used in skincare routines to promote lymphatic drainage and reduce facial puffiness.

CHAPTER ONE

HISTORICAL CONTEXT

A. Origins And Evolution

Ancient China: Early Practices And Philosophies

Development Through Dynasties (Han, Tang, Ming, Qing)

B. Influences And Adaptations

Impact On Neighboring Cultures (Korea, Japan, Vietnam)

Integration Into Western Practices

1. Ancient China: Early Practices and Philosophies

Early Practices: The origins of Gua Sha can be traced back to early Chinese civilizations, where various scraping techniques were used to treat ailments and maintain health. In these early practices, everyday objects like spoons or pieces of smooth stone were used to scrape the skin, promoting circulation and releasing toxins.

Philosophical Foundations: The practice of Gua Sha is rooted in the philosophical and medical principles of Traditional Chinese Medicine (TCM). Key concepts include:

Qi (Vital Energy): TCM posits that qi flows through meridians (energy channels) in the body. Gua Sha aims to remove blockages and improve the flow of qi.

Blood Circulation: The practice is also based on the idea that proper blood circulation is essential for health. Gua Sha is thought to invigorate blood flow and reduce stagnation.

Balance and Harmony: TCM emphasizes the balance of yin and yang, as well as the harmony between the body's internal organs and external factors. Gua Sha helps to restore balance by addressing areas of stagnation and imbalance.

2. Development Through Dynasties

Han Dynasty (206 BCE – 220 CE):

During the Han Dynasty, Gua Sha was formalized as part of medical practice. Medical texts from this period, such as the "Huangdi Neijing" (Yellow Emperor's Inner Canon), outline the use of scraping techniques for various health conditions.

The Han Dynasty also saw the development of more sophisticated tools and techniques for Gua Sha, and the practice became more standardized.

Tang Dynasty (618 – 907 CE):

The Tang Dynasty is noted for its advancements in Chinese medicine, including Gua Sha. During this period, the practice was further refined and documented in medical texts.

The Tang Dynasty also saw an increase in the use of specialized Gua Sha tools, and the practice spread to other regions of Asia.

Ming Dynasty (1368 – 1644 CE):

The Ming Dynasty brought significant developments in medical literature and practice. Gua Sha continued to be a part of medical treatments, and its techniques were detailed in various medical texts.

The Ming period also saw the introduction of Gua Sha into mainstream health practices, and it began to be more widely practiced among the general population.

Qing Dynasty (1644 – 1912 CE):

The Qing Dynasty saw the continuation and consolidation of Gua Sha practices. This period witnessed the use of Gua Sha in various therapeutic settings, including clinics and households.

The Qing Dynasty's medical texts further elaborated on the technique, its benefits, and its applications for different ailments.

B. Influences and Adaptations

1. Impact on Neighboring Cultures

Korea:

In Korea, Gua Sha is known as "Sujeok" or "Sujeong." The practice was influenced by Chinese medicine and adapted to local customs and health practices.

Korean Gua Sha often involves similar scraping techniques and tools, but with some regional variations in methodology and application.

Japan:

In Japan, Gua Sha is known as "Sokushi." The practice was introduced through Chinese influence and has been integrated into Japanese traditional medicine.

Japanese adaptations may include variations in techniques and tools, with a focus on specific health conditions relevant to Japanese cultural practices.

Vietnam:

In Vietnam, Gua Sha is known as "Cạo Gió." The practice has been adapted to Vietnamese traditional medicine, with its own regional variations in techniques and cultural significance.

Cạo Gió is widely used in Vietnam for various ailments, particularly for colds and muscle pain, reflecting the integration of Gua Sha into Vietnamese health practices.

2. Integration into Western Practices

Introduction to the West:

Gua Sha began gaining attention in Western countries in the late 20th and early 21st centuries. Initially introduced through alternative medicine and holistic health communities, it was recognized for its potential benefits.

Western practitioners and researchers have increasingly explored Gua Sha's applications for pain relief, muscle tension, and other health issues.

Modern Adaptations:

In the West, Gua Sha has been adapted and integrated into various wellness practices. For example, Gua Sha tools made of jade or rose quartz are popular in skincare routines, where they are used to promote lymphatic drainage and reduce facial puffiness.

The practice has been validated by some modern research, which has led to its incorporation into physical therapy and holistic health approaches.

Cultural Exchange:

The integration of Gua Sha into Western practices reflects broader trends in cultural exchange and the increasing acceptance of traditional and complementary therapies.

Gua Sha's growing popularity in the West demonstrates a blending of traditional Chinese medicine with modern health and wellness trends.

THE THEORY BEHIND GUASHA

A. Traditional Chinese Medicine Principles

Qi (Energy) And Blood Flow

Meridian Systems And Acupoints

B. Guasha Tools And Techniques

Materials Used (Jade, Horn, Plastic, Etc.)

Common Techniques And Their Purposes

A. Traditional Chinese Medicine Principles

1. Qi (Energy) and Blood Flow

Qi (Vital Energy):

In Traditional Chinese Medicine (TCM), Qi is considered the vital energy that flows through the body, essential for maintaining health and vitality. It circulates through pathways known as meridians, which are akin to channels or highways of energy.

Qi is responsible for various physiological functions, including the regulation of body temperature, digestion, and immune response. Disruptions or blockages in the flow of Qi can lead to illness or discomfort.

Blood Flow:

Blood in TCM is closely related to Qi and is essential for nourishing and sustaining the body. Blood flow supports the distribution of nutrients and removal of waste products.

Proper blood circulation is believed to help maintain health and prevent disease. Stagnation of blood, which can occur due to physical injury, stress, or poor lifestyle, is thought to contribute to various ailments.

Gua Sha's Role:

Gua Sha is based on the principle of improving the flow of Qi and blood. By scraping the skin, Gua Sha aims to stimulate circulation, remove blockages, and enhance the body's natural healing processes.

The technique is believed to invigorate blood flow, disperse stagnation, and promote the movement of Qi throughout the body.

2. Meridian Systems and AcuPoints

Meridian Systems:

The meridian system is a network of channels through which Qi and blood flow. In TCM, there are 12 primary meridians, each corresponding to specific organs and functions.

These meridians connect various parts of the body, and imbalances or blockages in these pathways can affect overall health.

AcuPoints (Acupuncture Points):

AcuPoints are specific locations along the meridians where Qi is believed to be concentrated or influenced. Stimulation of these points can affect the flow of Qi and help balance the body's energy.

Gua Sha targets areas on the skin that correspond to specific meridians and acuPoints. By applying pressure and scraping along these areas, the technique aims to enhance Qi flow and address imbalances.

Gua Sha's Application:

During a Gua Sha session, the practitioner may focus on specific meridians or acuPoints depending on the patient's condition. The scraping motion is believed to stimulate these points and improve the flow of Qi and blood.

B. Gua Sha Tools and Techniques
1. Materials Used

Jade:

Jade is a traditional material used in Gua Sha tools. It is prized for its smooth texture and cooling properties. In TCM, jade is believed to have healing and balancing qualities.

Jade tools are often used for facial Gua Sha, where their smooth surface is thought to promote lymphatic drainage and enhance skin health.

Horn:

Historically, tools made from buffalo horn or other animal horns were used in Gua Sha. Horn tools are valued for their durability and smooth scraping surface.

Horn tools are less common today but are still used in some traditional practices.

Plastic:

Plastic Gua Sha tools are more modern and are often designed to be lightweight and easy to clean. They are used for both facial and body Gua Sha.

Plastic tools are typically affordable and come in various shapes and sizes, catering to different areas of the body.

Other Materials:

Other materials such as stainless steel, glass, and rose quartz are also used in Gua Sha tools. Each material offers different benefits and feels on the skin.

2. Common Techniques and Their Purposes

Scraping (Gua):

Technique: The primary technique involves using a smooth-edged tool to scrape the skin in long, firm strokes. The scraping is typically done along the direction of the muscle fibers and meridians.

Purpose: This technique is used to stimulate circulation, release muscle tension, and promote the flow of Qi and blood. It can also help in reducing pain and improving flexibility.

Pressing:

Technique: Pressing involves applying steady, moderate pressure with the Gua Sha tool on specific areas or acuPoints.

Purpose: This technique is used to target deeper layers of muscle and connective tissue, providing relief from chronic pain and improving local circulation.

Brushing:

Technique: Brushing involves using a gentle, sweeping motion over the skin, often with a lighter touch than scraping.

Purpose: Brushing is typically used for sensitive areas or the face, where the goal is to promote lymphatic drainage, reduce puffiness, and enhance skin health.

Petrissage:

Technique: Petrissage involves kneading or pinching the skin and underlying tissues using the Gua Sha tool.

Purpose: This technique aims to relax muscle tension, improve circulation, and break down adhesions in the muscles.

Combination Techniques:

Technique: Practitioners may combine various techniques depending on the patient's needs and the area being treated.

Purpose: The combination of techniques allows for a comprehensive approach to addressing different aspects of a condition, enhancing overall therapeutic effects.

CHAPTER TWO

THE PRACTICE OF GUASHA

A. Preparing For Guasha

Setting Up The Environment

Choosing Appropriate Tools And Techniques

B. Step-By-Step Guide

Detailed Instructions For Self-Care

Professional Practice And What To Expect

C. Common Areas Of Application

Neck And Shoulders

Back And Legs

Face And Scalp

A. Preparing for Gua Sha

1. Setting Up the Environment

Cleanliness: Ensure that the environment is clean and hygienic. This helps prevent infections and ensures a comfortable experience. Clean the Gua Sha tools before and after each use.

Comfort: Create a comfortable setting by using a clean, soft surface, such as a massage table or a cushioned chair. Ensure the room is warm and well-ventilated to enhance relaxation.

Lighting and Atmosphere: Soft, ambient lighting and calming music can help set a soothing atmosphere, making the experience more pleasant and relaxing.

Accessibility: Make sure the area being treated is easily accessible. If treating the back or other hard-to-reach areas, have someone assist you or use a mirror to guide the application.

2. Choosing Appropriate Tools and Techniques

Tools: Select a Gua Sha tool based on the area being treated and personal preference. Common materials include jade, rose quartz, stainless steel, or plastic.

Jade Tools: Ideal for facial Gua Sha due to their smooth texture and cooling properties.

Stainless Steel Tools: Durable and easy to clean; suitable for both body and facial use.

Plastic Tools: Lightweight and versatile; suitable for various areas but may lack the traditional feel of stone tools.

Techniques: Choose techniques based on the condition being addressed and the area of the body.

Scraping: For general circulation improvement and muscle tension relief.

Pressing: For deeper muscle relief or targeting specific acuPoints.

Brushing: For sensitive areas or facial Gua Sha.

Combination: Using multiple techniques for comprehensive treatment.

B. Step-by-Step Guide

1. Detailed Instructions for Self-Care

Preparation:

Cleanse: Start by cleansing the skin where Gua Sha will be applied. This helps remove any impurities and allows for better tool movement.

Apply Lubricant: Apply a thin layer of massage oil or moisturizer to the skin.

This reduces friction and helps the tool glide smoothly.

Self-Care Steps:

Positioning: Sit or lie down comfortably. Ensure that the area being treated is accessible and relaxed.

Scraping Technique:

Hold the Gua Sha tool at a 30-45 degree angle to the skin.

Use firm but gentle pressure to scrape the skin in long, smooth strokes, following the direction of the muscle fibers or meridian lines.

Repeat the scraping motion 4-6 times on each area, adjusting pressure as needed.

Post-Treatment: After the session, gently cleanse the skin to remove any residual oil. Apply a soothing lotion if needed. Rest and hydrate to support the body's natural healing process.

Frequency: For self-care, Gua Sha can be performed 2-3 times a week. Monitor how your body responds and adjust the frequency accordingly.

2. Professional Practice and What to Expect

Initial Consultation:

A professional Gua Sha session usually begins with a consultation where the practitioner will assess your health, discuss your concerns, and determine the appropriate treatment plan.

During the Session:

Assessment: The practitioner will assess the areas of tension or discomfort and choose the appropriate tools and techniques.

Technique: The practitioner will use their expertise to apply Gua Sha with controlled pressure and precise movements, targeting specific areas and acuPoints.

Comfort: Communicate with the practitioner about your comfort level and any pain or discomfort during the session. They can adjust the technique and pressure as needed.

Post-Treatment Care:

After the session, you may experience mild redness or bruising, which is normal and typically resolves within a few days.

Follow any post-treatment recommendations from the practitioner, such as hydration or rest. They may also provide guidance on self-care and future treatments.

C. Common Areas of Application

1. Neck and Shoulders

Purpose: Gua Sha is commonly used on the neck and shoulders to relieve tension, reduce stiffness, and improve circulation.

Technique:

Use long, upward strokes from the base of the neck to the shoulders.

Apply moderate pressure to target muscle knots and areas of tightness.

Adjust the angle and pressure based on sensitivity and comfort.

2. Back and Legs

Purpose: The back and legs are frequently treated to alleviate muscle soreness, improve blood flow, and release accumulated tension.

Technique:

For the back, use broad strokes from the lower back to the upper back, following the muscle lines.

For the legs, apply long strokes from the thighs to the calves, focusing on areas of muscle tension or tightness.

Ensure that you use enough lubricant to reduce friction and make the scraping more comfortable.

3. Face and Scalp

Purpose: Gua Sha on the face and scalp can enhance circulation, reduce puffiness, and improve skin tone.

Technique:

Face: Use gentle, upward strokes, starting from the center of the face and moving outward. Focus on areas like the jawline, cheeks, and forehead.

Scalp: Apply gentle pressure with circular motions to stimulate blood flow and relax the scalp. This can also help with tension headaches.

Tools: Use smooth, rounded tools like jade rollers or smaller Gua Sha tools designed for facial use.

BENEFITS AND EFFECTS

A. Physiological Benefits

Improved Circulation

Pain Relief And Muscle Relaxation

B. Psychological And Emotional Benefits

Stress Reduction

Enhanced Overall Well-Being

C. Case Studies And Anecdotes

Personal Stories And Testimonials

Clinical Observations And Research Findings

A. Physiological Benefits

1. Improved Circulation

Mechanism: Gua Sha enhances circulation by stimulating blood flow to the treated areas. The scraping action creates micro-trauma to the skin and underlying tissues, which triggers the body's natural healing response and increases blood flow.

Effects:

Local Circulation: Increased blood flow helps deliver more oxygen and nutrients to the muscles and tissues, aiding in their repair and recovery.

Systemic Effects: Enhanced local circulation can contribute to overall improved blood flow, which can be beneficial for general health and vitality.

Detoxification: Improved circulation helps flush out metabolic waste products and toxins from the body, promoting detoxification.

2. Pain Relief and Muscle Relaxation

Mechanism: Gua Sha helps relieve pain and relax muscles by breaking up adhesions and reducing muscle tension. The technique can also stimulate the release of endorphins, which are natural painkillers.

Effects:

Reduced Pain: By alleviating muscle tension and increasing blood flow, Gua Sha can help reduce pain, particularly in areas affected by chronic muscle soreness, stiffness, or tension.

Muscle Relaxation: The technique promotes relaxation of tight muscles and can improve range of motion, making it beneficial for conditions like back pain, neck stiffness, and sore muscles.

Inflammation Reduction: Gua Sha can help reduce inflammation by promoting better circulation and dispersing stagnant blood, which can be particularly useful for inflammatory conditions.

B. Psychological and Emotional Benefits

1. Stress Reduction

Mechanism: Gua Sha can contribute to stress reduction by promoting relaxation and calming the nervous system. The physical sensation of the scraping, along with the overall therapeutic experience, helps reduce stress levels.

Effects:

Relaxation Response: The gentle pressure and rhythmic movement of Gua Sha can induce a relaxation response, helping to lower cortisol levels (the stress hormone).

Mental Calmness: The soothing nature of the treatment can help clear the mind and promote a sense of calm, which is beneficial for managing stress and anxiety.

2. Enhanced Overall Well-Being

Mechanism: Regular Gua Sha treatments can support overall well-being by enhancing both physical and emotional health. The practice helps integrate the body's physical and energetic systems, contributing to a holistic sense of health.

Effects:

Improved Mood: By relieving physical discomfort and promoting relaxation,

Gua Sha can positively impact mood and emotional state.

Greater Vitality: Enhanced circulation and reduced muscle tension contribute to improved energy levels and a greater sense of vitality.

Holistic Balance: Gua Sha supports the balance of Qi and blood flow, which aligns with TCM principles of health and can foster a sense of overall well-being.

C. Case Studies and Anecdotes

1. Personal Stories and Testimonials

Personal Accounts: Many individuals who have undergone Gua Sha report significant improvements in their health and well-being. Testimonials often highlight benefits such as reduced muscle pain, increased flexibility, and improved skin appearance.

Example: A person with chronic neck pain might share how Gua Sha provided relief from stiffness and discomfort, allowing them to move more freely and experience less daily pain.

Example: Someone who has used Gua Sha for facial treatments might note improvements in skin tone, reduced puffiness, and a more youthful appearance.

2. Clinical Observations and Research Findings

Clinical Observations: Healthcare practitioners have observed positive effects of Gua Sha in various clinical settings. These observations often align with traditional claims, such as reduced pain and improved circulation.

Example: Observations in physical therapy clinics might show that patients receiving Gua Sha treatment report less muscle soreness and quicker recovery times compared to those who did not receive the treatment.

Research Findings: Scientific research on Gua Sha is growing, with studies providing evidence for its efficacy in various applications.

Example: A study published in the journal *Pain Medicine* found that Gua Sha was effective in reducing pain and improving range of motion in patients with chronic neck pain.

Example: Research in *The Journal of Alternative and Complementary Medicine* has indicated that Gua Sha can significantly improve circulation and reduce muscle pain, supporting traditional claims about its benefits.

CHAPTER THREE

ADDRESSING MISCONCEPTIONS

A. Myths Vs. Facts

Common Misconceptions Debunked

Evidence-Based Clarifications

B. Potential Risks And Precautions

Safety Guidelines

Contraindications And When To Avoid

A. Myths vs. Facts

1. Common Misconceptions Debunked

Myth: Gua Sha is Painful and Bruising is Harmful

Fact: While Gua Sha involves scraping the skin, it should not be excessively painful.

Mild bruising or redness, known as "sha," is a normal response and typically fades within a few days. The bruising is generally a sign of increased blood flow and the body's natural healing process. However, if the pain is severe or if there is significant, prolonged bruising, it may indicate too much pressure or an improper technique.

Myth: Gua Sha is Only for Muscle Pain Relief

Fact: Although Gua Sha is widely used for muscle pain relief, its benefits extend beyond this. It is also used to improve circulation, support immune function, and enhance skin health. In TCM, it is applied to balance Qi and blood flow throughout the body, which can impact various aspects of health.

Myth: Gua Sha is Only Effective with Specific Tools

Fact: While traditional tools like jade or horn are commonly used, Gua Sha can be performed with various materials such as plastic or stainless steel. The effectiveness of Gua Sha is more dependent on technique and application rather than the specific tool used. The choice of tool can, however, influence comfort and specific benefits.

Myth: Gua Sha is a New Trend in Wellness

Fact: Gua Sha is a traditional practice with roots dating back thousands of years in Chinese medicine. Its resurgence in recent years is due to a growing interest in holistic and complementary therapies, but its principles and techniques have been practiced and refined over millennia.

Myth: Gua Sha Can Replace Medical Treatments

Fact: Gua Sha is a complementary therapy that can enhance overall well-being and support conventional medical treatments. It should not replace medical advice or treatment for serious conditions. Always consult with a healthcare provider for medical concerns or before starting new treatments.

2. Evidence-Based Clarifications

Evidence on Pain Relief: Studies have shown that Gua Sha can be effective for pain relief and muscle relaxation. Research published in *Pain Medicine* demonstrated that Gua Sha improved pain and range of motion in patients with chronic neck pain, supporting its use for musculoskeletal issues.

Evidence on Circulation: Evidence from studies, including those published in *The Journal of Alternative and Complementary Medicine*, supports the claim that Gua Sha enhances circulation. This is consistent with the traditional belief that it stimulates blood flow and promotes healing.

Evidence on Safety: Research indicates that Gua Sha is generally safe when performed correctly. Most reported side effects are mild and include temporary redness or bruising. Serious adverse effects are rare and often associated with improper technique or pre-existing conditions.

B. Potential Risks and Precautions

1. Safety Guidelines

Proper Technique: To minimize risks, it is important to use correct Gua Sha techniques. This includes applying appropriate pressure and using a tool with a smooth, rounded edge to avoid skin damage.

Clean Tools: Ensure that Gua Sha tools are thoroughly cleaned before and after each use to prevent infections and maintain hygiene.

Skin Preparation: Always apply a suitable lubricant (such as massage oil or cream) to the skin before performing Gua Sha to reduce friction and prevent irritation.

Gentle Approach: Start with light pressure and gradually increase as needed. Excessive pressure can lead to more severe bruising and discomfort.

2. Contraindications and When to Avoid

Skin Conditions: Avoid Gua Sha on areas with open wounds, rashes, or infections. The scraping action could exacerbate these conditions or lead to further irritation.

Medical Conditions: Individuals with certain medical conditions, such as bleeding disorders, severe heart conditions, or recent surgeries, should avoid Gua Sha or consult a healthcare provider before using it. This is particularly important for those with conditions that affect blood clotting or skin integrity.

Pregnancy: Gua Sha may not be recommended during pregnancy, especially on the abdomen or lower back. Consult a healthcare provider to ensure it is safe to use during pregnancy.

Recent Injuries: Avoid Gua Sha on recent injuries or areas with acute inflammation. It may exacerbate pain or swelling in these cases.

INTEGRATION WITH MODERN PRACTICES

A. Guasha In Contemporary Wellness

Usage In Spas And Wellness Centers

Integration With Other Therapies
(Acupuncture, Massage)

B. Guasha In Daily Life

Incorporating Into A Wellness Routine

Adaptations For Different Lifestyles
And Needs

A. Gua Sha in Contemporary Wellness

1. Usage in Spas and Wellness Centers

Spa Treatments:

Facial Gua Sha: Many spas offer facial Gua Sha as part of their skincare treatments. This involves using smooth-edged tools, often made of jade or rose quartz, to enhance lymphatic drainage, reduce puffiness, and improve skin tone and texture.

Body Gua Sha: Some wellness centers incorporate Gua Sha into their body treatments to address muscle tension, improve circulation, and promote relaxation. This can be part of a larger therapeutic session that includes massage or other bodywork techniques.

Benefits in Spa Settings:

Relaxation: Gua Sha is used to create a calming and restorative experience, helping clients relax and unwind.

Enhanced Skin Health: In facial treatments, Gua Sha is believed to promote collagen production, reduce the appearance of fine lines, and improve overall skin radiance.

Comprehensive Care: Spa settings often combine Gua Sha with other wellness practices, such as aromatherapy or hot stone therapy, to provide a holistic treatment experience.

2. Integration with Other Therapies

Acupuncture:

Complementary Therapy: Gua Sha is often used alongside acupuncture to enhance the effects of treatment. While acupuncture targets specific points to regulate Qi and blood flow, Gua Sha can be applied to broader areas to relieve muscle tension and improve circulation.

Synergistic Effects: Combining Gua Sha with acupuncture can provide a more comprehensive approach to addressing various health issues, such as chronic pain, stress, and musculoskeletal problems.

Massage Therapy:

Enhanced Outcomes: Gua Sha can be integrated into massage therapy sessions to deepen the benefits of manual therapy. The scraping action can help to release muscle knots and improve blood flow, enhancing the overall effectiveness of the massage.

Sequential Use: Gua Sha is sometimes used as a preliminary treatment to prepare the muscles for deeper massage work. The increased circulation and muscle relaxation can make subsequent massage techniques more effective.

Other Therapies:

Cupping Therapy: Gua Sha and cupping are both traditional therapies that can be used together to address muscle tension and improve circulation. Cupping creates suction to draw blood to the surface, while Gua Sha helps to disperse stagnation and enhance overall circulation.

Yoga and Stretching: Incorporating Gua Sha into a wellness routine that includes yoga or stretching can support muscle recovery, improve flexibility, and enhance the benefits of these practices.

B. Gua Sha in Daily Life

1. Incorporating into a Wellness Routine

Self-Care Practice:

Daily Routine: Gua Sha can be incorporated into a daily wellness routine, particularly for facial care. For example, a few minutes of Gua Sha in the morning or evening can help with lymphatic drainage, reduce puffiness, and promote relaxation.

Body Care: For body care, Gua Sha can be performed a few times a week to address areas of muscle tension or soreness. It can be especially beneficial after exercise or long periods of sitting.

Guided Routine:

Techniques: Follow a structured routine that includes specific techniques and areas to focus on. For facial Gua Sha, this might involve gentle strokes from the center of the face outward. For body Gua Sha, use longer strokes along the muscle lines.

Tools and Products: Use appropriate tools and products, such as facial oils or body lotions, to enhance the effectiveness of the practice. Ensure tools are clean and well-maintained.

2. Adaptations for Different Lifestyles and Needs

Busy Lifestyles:

Quick Sessions: For those with busy schedules, short, targeted Gua Sha sessions can be effective. Focus on specific areas, such as the neck or face, for a few minutes to achieve benefits without a significant time commitment.

Portable Tools: Use compact and travel-friendly Gua Sha tools that can be easily carried and used on the go.

Active Lifestyles:

Post-Exercise Recovery: Gua Sha can be adapted as part of a post-exercise recovery routine. Use it to relieve muscle soreness and stiffness, enhance circulation, and support quicker recovery.

Integration with Stretching: Combine Gua Sha with stretching exercises to improve flexibility and overall muscle function.

Sensitive Skin:

Gentle Techniques: For individuals with sensitive skin, use lighter pressure and smooth, rounded tools. Avoid areas with skin conditions or irritation.

Soothing Products: Use hypoallergenic or soothing oils and lotions to prevent irritation and enhance the comfort of the Gua Sha practice.

Health Conditions:

Consultation: Individuals with specific health conditions should consult with a healthcare provider before incorporating Gua Sha into their routine. This is particularly important for those with chronic conditions or injuries that might be affected by the practice.

CHAPTER FOUR

CULTURAL AND PERSONAL REFLECTIONS

A. Guasha In Personal Journeys

Personal Reflections And Transformations

Stories From Practitioners And Patients

B. Cultural Significance

Symbolism And Cultural Narratives

Guasha's Role In Preserving Cultural Heritage

A. Gua Sha in Personal Journeys

1.   Personal   Reflections   and Transformations

Personal Transformation:

Physical Benefits: Many individuals who incorporate Gua Sha into their wellness routines report significant improvements in their physical health. For some, the practice has led to reduced muscle pain, increased flexibility, and improved overall energy levels.

Emotional Growth: Gua Sha often facilitates a deeper connection to one's body and self. The practice can offer moments of mindfulness and introspection, leading to a greater awareness of physical and emotional states.

Routine Integration: For some, integrating Gua Sha into daily or weekly routines becomes a transformative ritual. This regular practice can foster a sense of discipline and self-care, enhancing overall well-being and personal satisfaction.

Challenges and Adaptations:

Learning Curve: Initially, practitioners may face challenges in mastering the technique or adapting the practice to their needs. Over time, many find that overcoming these challenges contributes to personal growth and a deeper appreciation for Gua Sha.

Adaptation to Lifestyle: Individuals with busy or varied lifestyles often adapt Gua Sha practices to fit their schedules. These adaptations might include shorter sessions, different techniques, or combining Gua Sha with other wellness practices.

2. Stories from Practitioners and Patients

Practitioners' Stories:

Personal Anecdotes: Practitioners often share how Gua Sha has become a valuable part of their professional practice. Many report that integrating Gua Sha with other therapies, such as acupuncture or massage, enhances their ability to help clients achieve better outcomes.

Professional Growth: For some practitioners, the journey with Gua Sha involves continuous learning and adaptation. They might describe how studying and applying Gua Sha has deepened their understanding of holistic health and broadened their therapeutic skills.

Patients' Stories:

Success Stories: Patients frequently recount positive experiences with Gua Sha, such as significant relief from chronic pain, improved skin conditions, or better stress management. These stories often highlight the personalized benefits they've received from the practice.

Transformational Experiences: Some patients share how Gua Sha has transformed their approach to wellness. For example, those who struggled with stress or muscular issues may find that regular Gua Sha sessions become a vital part of their self-care routines, leading to improved quality of life.

B. Cultural Significance

1. Symbolism and Cultural Narratives

Traditional Symbolism:

Healing and Balance: In Traditional Chinese Medicine (TCM), Gua Sha symbolizes the balance of Qi (energy) and the flow of blood. The practice reflects the cultural belief in harmonizing the body's internal energies to maintain health and prevent disease.

Holistic Health: Gua Sha is part of a broader cultural narrative that emphasizes holistic health and the interconnectedness of physical, emotional, and spiritual well-being.

Cultural Narratives:

Historical Roots: Gua Sha has deep historical roots in Chinese culture, often linked to ancient practices and philosophies. It is part of a rich tapestry of traditional therapies that have been passed down through generations.

Cultural Continuity: The practice of Gua Sha reflects a continuity of cultural traditions and medical knowledge. It embodies the preservation of traditional healing arts within modern contexts, bridging ancient wisdom with contemporary wellness practices.

2. Gua Sha's Role in Preserving Cultural Heritage

Preservation of Tradition:

Traditional Practices: Gua Sha helps preserve traditional Chinese healing practices and philosophies. By maintaining and adapting these practices, practitioners and enthusiasts contribute to the ongoing legacy of Chinese medicine.

Cultural Education: Modern interest in Gua Sha often includes educational efforts to inform others about its historical and cultural significance. This helps preserve knowledge and understanding of traditional techniques and their cultural contexts.

Global Influence:

Cultural Exchange: As Gua Sha gains popularity outside of China, it becomes a vehicle for cultural exchange. This global awareness helps preserve the practice by introducing it to new audiences while respecting its traditional roots.

Adaptation and Innovation: The adaptation of Gua Sha in different cultural settings allows for innovation while honoring its traditional origins. This dynamic interaction helps ensure that

Gua Sha remains relevant and respected in diverse contexts.

FUTURE DIRECTIONS

A. Evolving Practices And Research

Emerging Trends And Innovations

Ongoing Research And Studies

B. Expanding Awareness

Educational Initiatives And Workshops

Global Recognition And Acceptance

A. Evolving Practices and Research

1. Emerging Trends and Innovations

Technological Integration:

Advanced Tools: The development of new materials and designs for Gua Sha tools, such as ergonomic handles or tools made from advanced materials like stainless steel or silicone, is enhancing comfort and effectiveness.

Digital Integration: The use of apps and digital platforms to guide Gua Sha practices is increasing. These platforms may offer instructional videos, tracking features, and personalized recommendations based on user needs.

Combination Therapies:

Integrated Approaches: There is a growing trend to combine Gua Sha with other modern wellness practices, such as biofeedback, infrared therapy, or cryotherapy, to amplify its benefits. These combinations aim to create synergistic effects for enhanced therapeutic outcomes.

Customization: Advances in personalized medicine are influencing Gua Sha practices, with an emphasis on tailoring treatments to individual health profiles and needs, potentially integrating genetic or biometric data to optimize results.

Enhanced Product Lines:

Cosmetic Innovations: The use of Gua Sha in cosmetic products is expanding, including tools designed for facial treatments with features such as cooling effects or integrated massagers to enhance skincare routines.

DIY Kits: There is a rise in DIY Gua Sha kits for home use, including pre-packaged sets with tools, instructional materials, and complementary skincare products.

2. Ongoing Research and Studies

Clinical Trials:

Scientific Validation: Ongoing clinical trials are focusing on scientifically validating the benefits of Gua Sha for various health conditions, such as chronic pain, muscle recovery, and skin health. These studies aim to provide empirical evidence to support traditional claims and refine techniques.

Longitudinal Studies: Researchers are conducting longitudinal studies to assess the long-term effects of Gua Sha on overall health and well-being, examining its efficacy over extended periods and its impact on chronic conditions.

Mechanistic Research:

Physiological Mechanisms: Studies are exploring the physiological mechanisms underlying Gua Sha, such as how it influences microcirculation, cellular repair processes, and the body's inflammatory response.

Comparative Studies: Research comparing Gua Sha to other therapeutic modalities, such as acupuncture or physical therapy, aims to understand its relative effectiveness and potential benefits when used in combination with other treatments.

B. Expanding Awareness

1. Educational Initiatives and Workshops

Training Programs:

Professional Development: The development of formal training programs and certifications for practitioners is increasing. These programs often include comprehensive education on Gua Sha techniques, safety protocols, and integration with other therapies.

Community Workshops: Workshops and seminars aimed at the general public are becoming more common. These educational events focus on teaching the basics of Gua Sha, its benefits, and practical application for self-care.

Online Resources:

Digital Education: Online courses, webinars, and tutorials are expanding access to Gua Sha education. These resources provide information on technique, safety, and benefits to a global audience, making it easier for individuals to learn and apply Gua Sha practices.

Content Creation: Influencers and experts in the wellness community are creating content that promotes Gua Sha, including blogs, social media posts, and video demonstrations, which contribute to raising awareness and educating the public.

2. Global Recognition and Acceptance

Cross-Cultural Integration:

Cultural Exchange: Gua Sha's popularity is growing globally, leading to increased cultural exchange and integration into various wellness practices. This broader acceptance helps to foster a deeper understanding of Gua Sha's origins and applications.

Collaborative Practices: International collaborations between practitioners and researchers are enhancing the understanding and application of Gua Sha across different cultural and medical contexts.

Institutional Endorsement:

Healthcare Integration: There is a growing recognition of Gua Sha within conventional healthcare settings. Some healthcare providers and integrative medicine clinics are beginning to incorporate Gua Sha into their treatment protocols, acknowledging its benefits and potential.

Academic Research: Increased academic interest and research into Gua Sha are contributing to its acceptance in the scientific and medical communities. Publications in peer-reviewed journals and presentations at conferences are raising the profile of Gua Sha as a credible therapeutic modality.

CONCLUSION

A. Summary Of Key Points

Recap Of Guasha's Significance And Benefits

B. Final Thoughts

Encouragement For Readers To Explore And Experience Guasha

A. Summary of Key Points

Significance of Gua Sha: Gua Sha is a traditional Chinese healing practice with deep historical roots, dating back thousands of years. It is a technique involving scraping the skin with a smooth-edged tool to stimulate circulation, promote healing, and balance Qi (energy) in the body. This practice reflects broader TCM principles, emphasizing the interconnectedness of body, mind, and spirit.

Benefits of Gua Sha:

Physiological Benefits: Gua Sha enhances blood circulation, reduces muscle tension, and alleviates pain. The technique promotes muscle relaxation, aids in detoxification, and supports overall physical health.

Psychological and Emotional Benefits: It can help reduce stress, promote relaxation, and contribute to an improved sense of well-being. The practice fosters a holistic approach to health that encompasses both physical and emotional dimensions.

Cultural and Personal Reflections: Gua Sha is not only a therapeutic technique but also a significant cultural practice. It embodies traditional Chinese philosophies and has been integrated into modern wellness practices. Personal stories and cultural significance highlight its role in preserving traditional healing arts while adapting to contemporary needs.

Integration and Future Directions:

Modern Integration: Gua Sha is increasingly incorporated into contemporary wellness practices, including spas, and combined with other therapies like acupuncture and massage. Innovations in tools and techniques are enhancing its accessibility and effectiveness.

Research and Awareness: Ongoing research aims to validate Gua Sha's benefits and understand its mechanisms. Efforts to expand awareness through educational initiatives and global recognition are helping to integrate Gua Sha into broader wellness contexts.

B. Final Thoughts

Gua Sha offers a rich tapestry of benefits and cultural significance that extends beyond its traditional roots. Its integration into modern wellness practices demonstrates its enduring relevance and adaptability. As you explore Gua Sha, consider the following:

Explore Gua Sha: Whether you are seeking relief from physical discomfort, aiming to enhance your wellness routine, or interested in exploring traditional healing practices, Gua Sha provides a versatile and accessible tool for self-care.

Experience Gua Sha: Engaging in Gua Sha can be a deeply personal and transformative experience. Whether performed at home or in a professional setting, taking the time to learn and apply Gua Sha techniques can contribute to a greater sense of well-being and balance.

Stay Informed: As interest in Gua Sha grows, stay informed about new developments, research, and educational opportunities. This will help you make the most of this ancient practice and understand its evolving role in modern wellness.

By embracing Gua Sha and its benefits, you participate in a long-standing tradition of holistic health that continues

to enrich lives around the world.

END

www.ingramcontent.com/pod-product-compliance
Lightning Source LLC
Chambersburg PA
CBHW061059250726
48653CB00001B/473